Eating With

DIABETES

&

KIDNEY FAILURE

Diana Harvey Darrisaw

Welcome my name is Diana Harvey Darrisaw. I was able to share for over 35 years the complications that many patients went through eating with kidney failure and diabetes. Two conditions that are drawn to other. I know you can have healthy and happy meals if you are willing to sacrifice and be obedient to your needs. If you find what I share may help, **PLEASE MAKE NO ADVANCE STEPS UNTIL YOU DISCUSS IT WITH YOUR MEDICAL STAFF.**

Most of the things you read were based on my husband's experience with these conditions.

PROFESSIONALLY II WAS MENTORED BY WHO I SAW AS THE MASTER'S IN NUTRITION. I WAS EDUCATED ON AND OFF THE JOB IN THE FIELD OF WHAT SUPERVISING IN PATIENT NUTRITIONAL CARE WAS ALL ABOUT. I WAS EDUCATED AND CERTIFIED FROM NUTRITIONAL COURSES TAKEN AT PENN STATE AND GEORGIA STATE, I WORKED WITH PATIENTS DAILY FOR MANY YEARS, BUT IT STILL EFFECTED MY FAMILY. KIDNEY FAILURE AND DIABETES ARE VERY SERIOUS, AND EATING CORRECTLY IS AS IMPORTANT AS MEDICINE.

I AM NOT A MD OR DIETICIAN OR NUTRITIONIST, I WRITE FROM EXPERIENCES AND EDUCATION IN PATIENT CARE NUTRITION.

TO BE IN ANY FIELD OF WORK FOR OVER FORTY YEARS NON-STOP AND LEAVE WITH ANY KNOWLEDGE IS VERY SAD, I AM BLESSED WHAT I WAS ABLE TO ABSORB CONTINUE TO STAY 1955 UNTIL NOW AND FOR MANY MORE YEARS I PRAY.

MANY HEALTH CONDITIONS HAVE BEEN PASSED DOWN TO US, SO THIS MEANS WE HAVE A JOB ALREADY WAITING THAT WILL NEED DAILY ATTENTION AND SOMETIMES PHYSICAL CARE. EVERYONE RECEIVES THEIR BLESSINGS AND SAD TIMES. FOOD IS LIFE WHATEVER WAY IT IS DISTRIBUTED LIQUID OR SOLID, THE BEST IN NUTRITION EXPANDS LIFE AND GOOD CHOICES OF FOODS OFFER THIS.

TAKE THE TIME TO UNDERSTAND YOUR DIET WELL. I AM GOING TO GO THROUGH EACH   HEALTH-RELATED CONDITION. IN THIS WAY I FEEL UNDERSTANDING WILL BE MORE FAMILIAR. I WORKED FOR YEARS JUST WITH DIABETICS AND RENAL PATIENTS, THE OLD SCHOOL FORMAT WAS MUCH DIFFERENT WITH PATIENTS WITH KIDNEY FAILURE THEN IT IS NOW, I TAKE MY HAT OFF FOR THE RELEASE OF THE STRICTNESS FOR THE

PATIENTS WITH KIDNEY FAILURE. THE TERM RENAL IS THE NAME OF THE DIET YOU HAVE BEEN PUT ON. THE DIETS MUST BE FOLLOWED WITH AWESOME GUIDANCE AND UNDERSTANDING. EVERYONE IS GIVEN RULES ABOUT WHAT TO EAT AND NOT TO EAT. MANY CANNOT SEEM TO GET STARTED OR HAVE A ROUGH TIME STAYING ON TRACK.

ROBERT, MY HUSBAND, NEVER HAD A PROBLEM EATING SMILE. HE IS MORE STUBBORN THAN NOT KNOWING; NOTHING MAJOR, MY SON AND I KEPT HIM ON TRACK MEALTIMES, HE SAYS NOTHING, BUT HIS EXPRESSIONS TELL US PLEASE GIVE ME A BREAK. I HEARD THIS FROM THOUSANDS OF PATIENTS ALONG MY ROUGH JOURNEY. I AM USED TO IT. I WILL NOT BEND WHEN IT COMES TO HIM FOLLOWING HIS PROPER DIET,

THIS DIET RENAL TO ME IS AN EXCEEDINGLY DIFFICULT DIET BY ITSELF. IF YOU HAVE EATEN WHATEVER YOU DESIRED ALL YOUR LIFE CHANGES WILL AFFECT YOU, I INTEND TO KEEP MY SHARING REAL, BECAUSE THIS IS A REALITY THAT MUST BE AFFECTED EVERY DAY NOT JUST DURING THE WEEK AND WHEN THE WEEKEND COMES BACK TO THE OLD WAYS. EVERY DAY IT IS ALL ABOUT EXTENDING YOUR LIFE.

WHEN THE RULES ARE SET YOU MUST FOLLOW THEM. SOME ARE NOT WILLING TO ALLOW THEMSELVES TO ADJUST TO THE NEW MEAL PLAN. I FEEL THAT MANY REALLY DO NOT REALIZE HOW MUCH EATING PROPERLY PLAYS IN THEIR CONDITION. YOU FOLLOW YOUR MEDICAL STAFF DISCUSS AND TALK WITH THEM WHEN IN DOUBT.

My first direct contact with renal failure was when I was presented to check a renal lunch meal, I was responsible for reviewing the patient's food choices. My supervisor rewarded me with the job doing ALL renal diets for the next few years. I got better as time passed and gradually more patients were dealing with diabetes and renal meal planning.

When I was working no kind of potatoes or green leafy veggies, 40 grams of protein was only allowed for 3 meals, and you had better stick to it. My days were spent, checking menus patients filled out making sure they had not asked for or wrote anything that they should not have. Sometimes working on 20 to 25 renal diets also 20 combination diets. Old ways have their place in my life, As time moved on, new dietary discoveries came I accepted the new ways.

Let us have a good UNDERSTANDING in the term COMBINATION DIETS.

Any diet that addresses more than one condition. Simple right? Many of us have more than one health condition that calls for a dietary adjustment.

PLEASE LET YOUR MEDICAL TEAM be your leader in what you read, take nothing on your own when it comes to your health and well-being. I will repeat this often, this is serious to me.

I DO KNOW THERE ARE "FOLLOW THE LEADER" TYPE OF PEOPLE, ALTHOUGH WE ARE ALL GROWN UP.

HEALTH CARE ISSUES ARE IMPORTANT, THESE TWO DIETS ARE SPECIAL FOR ME MANY WE KNOW ARE GOING THROUGH SIMILAR HEALTH ISSUES. EACH HEALTH CONDITION IS RELATED IN SOME WAY TO THE NUTRITION WE GET. EVEN IF YOU JUST HAVE DIABETES OR JUST KIDNEY FAILURE, OR ON A TUBE FEEDING, YOU ARE STILL DEALING WITH SERIOUS MEAL PLANNING.

RECOGNIZE THE ERRORS IN YOUR MEAL PLANNING, THIS IS A DAILY PROCEDURE. BE AS UPDATED AS POSSIBLE IN THE UNDERSTANDING OF GRAMS AND MILIGRAMS WHEN READING FOOD LABELING. KNOW WHETHER IT MATTERS IF A FOOD IS 25 MILLIGRAMS (ABOUT THE WEIGHT OF A GRAIN OF RICE) OR 500 MILLIGRAMS (ABOUT HALF THE WEIGHT OF A SMALL PAPER CLIP) IT CAN HAVE A HUGE EFFECT. LIKE ANYTHING WE ARE NOT FAMILIAR WITH, IT IS JUST NOT UNDERSTANDABLE UNTIL WE LEARN WHAT IT IS ALL ABOUT. GUIDING MY HUSBAND IN WHAT HIS MEDICAL STAFF WANTS COMES A LITTLE EASIER FOR ME BECAUSE I WAS A PART OF IT FOR MANY YEARS.

I HAD A LENGTHY CAREER DEALING WITH THIS MATTER, I WAS ABLE TO STORE IT UNTIL IT WAS TIME TO BE USED AGAIN. THAT TIME IS NOW, NEVER DREAMING I WOULD USE IT FOR THE LOVE OF MY LIFE, MY HUSBAND.

RENAL AND DIABETES HAVE A PARTNERSHIP. IN THIS DIET EACH ONE MUST STAY IN ITS OWN CORNER BUT FORM AS ONE. AS I GO ALONG IT WILL BECOME CLEARER AND SENSIBLE WHERE I AM COMING FROM AND WHERE YOU CAN GO.

IN MY MEAL PLANNING THERE IS NO SIDE THAT TAKES THE MOST ATTENTION, BOTH ARE NEEDED AND SHOULD BE HANDLED WITH THE SAME THOUGHT IN MIND STAYING AS CLOSE TO THE GIVEN RULES AND THE CORRECT PORTION CONTROL.

YOU SHOULD FIND YOURSELVES PLANNING MEALS WITH FOODS BOTH WILL ENJOY AND CAN HAVE, AND THIS IS YOUR NEEDED WEAPON TO BRING BOTH DIETS TOGETHER, IF HE WANTS SHERBET AND YOU KNOW THE DIABETIC IS NOT ALLOWED THE SUGAR MOST HAVE, MAKE A SPECIAL CREAMY, COLD DESSERT USING A SUGAR SUBSTITUTE, THE RENAL SIDE IS USED TO IT, HOW? DIETS ARE DIFFERENT FOR THE SAME PERSON. SMILE.

DOES THE RENAL HAVE TO COUNT CALORIES OR WATCH HOW MUCH SUGAR? OR SALT? WELL IT IS LIKE THIS, CALORIES, CAN BE GOOD ENERGY FOR THE RENAL, SALT AND SODIUM SHOULD BE A RED FLAG MEANING NO. DIABETIC PARTNER A RED FLAG UP FOR ALL SUGARS, EXCEPT ARTIFICIAL SUGARS, ASK YOUR NUTRITION LEADER OR DOCTOR CONCERNING THE ABUNDANCE OF ALCOHOL SUGAR USED IN MANY FOODS NOW. SOME DIABETICS DO HAVE OTHER HEALTH CONDITIONS THAT DO RELATE TO FOODS SUCH AS CARDIO IN WHICH SODIUM AND SALTS ARE NO ALSO. IT CAN EXTREMELY HARD THESE DAYS TO FIND SOMEONE WITH JUST ONE HEALTH CONDITION RELATED TO EATING HABITS. WHATEVER YOU HAVE AND HAVE NOTS ARE JUST FOLLOW THEM CLOSELY.

AS YOU BEGIN YOUR MEAL PLANNING YOU WILL FIND THAT RED FLAGS ARE ALL OVER THE PLACE, WHY? THE DIET CALLS FOR IT. ROBERT SR. USED TO ALWAYS FUSS AND COMPLAIN ABOUT WHAT HE COULD NOT

HAVE IN TIME HE SUBSIDED IN WHAT HE HAD TO HAVE.

HOW SPECIAL IS OUR LIVES AND FAMILY ARE TO US USUALLY HELPS TO MAKE SURE WE DO IT RIGHT AS WE CAN. YES, I KNOW EASY SAID SHOULD BE EASILY DONE IT IS NOT. TO SIT AND TELL SOMEONE DO IT THIS WAY OR NO WAY, WHERE IS THE COMPASSION? LONG GONE, I GUESS. IN OUR HOME WE ALL TOGETHER DO WHAT IS BEST FOR THE PERSON IN NEED. I DO NOT KNOW WHAT IS OUT THERE, BUT MANY FEEL THE SAME AS I DO. YOU DO NOT HAVE TO BE A MEMBER OF THE SITUATION TO HAVE COMPASSION.

WE CANNOT GET AROUND THE FACT THAT BOTH CONDITIONS NEED ALL THAT IS RIGHT FOR THEM. OUR WAY IS PRAYER AND NEVER TO GIVE UP, JUST KEEP DOING YOUR BEST EVERYDAY, NO DAYS OFF. ROBERT SAYS THROUGH WHAT I AM GOING THROUGH AND SOMETHING COMES UP RIGHT I PASS ON TO ANOTHER IN HOPE THAT THEY CAN FIND THEIR WAY, AND THIS IS WHAT THIS BOOK IS ABOUT. RENALLY GET YOUR BLOOD CLEANED LIKE YOUR MEDICAL TEAM HAS APPOINTED, DO NOT MAKE THE MISTAKES IN, BECAUSE YOU FEEL BETTER WITHOUT DIAYLSIS. I HAVE NEVER SEEN SO MANY NEIGHBORHOOD DIALYSIS FACILITIES IN ONE AREA OF THE CITY. KIDNEY DISEASE IS ON THE MOVE BLOWING UP MORE EACH DAY. NO ONE HAS BEEN PROMISED WHAT THEIR FUTURE HOLDS, OR WHAT WILL HAPPEN MINUTE TO MINUTE OR DAY TO DAY, YOU WOULD THINK SO THE WAY THEY REACT TOWARD THOSE IN NEED, SORRY DOES NOT HELP OR HEAL, PRAYER AND LOVE DOES.

MY DEAR FRIEND DIED AND DID NOT EVEN TAKE AN ASPIRIN TABLET, NO PRIOR HISTORY OF ILLNESSES, WE

NEVER KNOW. WHAT YOU HAVE READ SO FAR GIVES AN IMPORTANT MESSAGE; DIABETES AND KIDNEY DISEASE ARE CONTROLLED BY WHAT IS EATEN. THERE ARE MANY, MANY TERMS I WOULD LIKE TO SHARE, I HAVE A RULE IN MY WRITING AND SHARING, STAYING AS CLOSE AS POSSIBLE TO MY OWN HOUSE SMILE. I AM NOT A DOCTOR IN ANY WAY. GIVE THE MEDICAL TEAMS ALL OVER FOR THEIR GUIDANCE AND HELP AND AWESOME BEDSIDE MANNER IF THEY ARE ANYTHING LIKE MY TEAM. I HAVE A GREAT DEAL OF EXPERIENCES IN WHAT I WRITE, I WAS THERE, SAW IT, DONE IT, AND TOOK ALL RESPONSIBILITIES CONNECTED TO WHATEVER IT WAS.

THE FOLLOWING HEALTH CONDITIONS YOU WILL FIND IN KIDNEY FAILURE ALSO. I AM SHARING THESE WITH YOU BECAUSE SOMEONE IS GOING THROUGH THESE ISSUES.

THESE ARE JUST EXAMPLES. CONSULT THE MEDICAL TEAM BEFORE DOING ANY DIET.

CARDIO/RENAL

DINNER

ROAST CHICKEN (NO SKIN)

SMOTHERED WHITE CABBAGE (ONIONS)

OVEN POTATOES/LOW SALT MARGARINE

SLICE WHITE BREAD/JAM

½ CUP WATER

4 OUNCES   FRUITED JELL O

No added sodium, potatoes should be soaked for at least 4 hours, do not serve chicken with skin, Season cabbage with a low cholesterol, unsaturated fat margarine, unsalted seasoning. Fluid is restricted so following your allowances close.

This is a healthy happy meal that always make room for happiness.

Just remember ALTHOUGH SOME VEGETABLES and FRUITS are ALLOWED, you must practice portion control. You will pick up that this combination diet, both diets are restricted from sodium or salt. This makes the meal planning easier.

GOUT/RENAL

BREAKFAST

½ CUP NATURAL CHERRY/PINEAPPLE JUICE

COOKED EGG

SLICE CINNO\MON TOAST

FAT-FREE CREAM CHEESE

½ CUP FLAVORED RICE MILK

4 OUNCES BREWED TEA /THIN SLICE OF FRESH LEMON

CHECK WHAT KIND OF HOT BEVERAGE THE DIET ALLOWS.

SINCE GOUT IS SERIOUS WITH PAIN FOLLOW THE RULES IN EATING CLOSE. USE A FLAVORING YOU ENJOY AND BE SURE YOU READ THE INGREDIENTS WELL. MAKING SURE THERE IS NOTHING OFFERED THAT YOU SHOULD NOT HAVE.

I HAVE FOUND MANY SENIORS HESITATE TO ASK QUESTIONS AND FOLLOW THE ANSWERS WHEN IT COMES TO HEALTH ISSUES. THIS WAS THE ATTITUDE DECADES AGO, THIS IS A NEW TIME, LISTEN AND FOLLOW IT IS ALL ABOUT YOU.

IF YOU HAVE A NEED FOR LEMON FOR TEA OR OTHER FOOD, USE A SMALL AMOUNT IF THIS IS NOT POSSIBLE (DON'T USE). YOU MUST KEEP AROUND THE CLOCK SELF-CONTROL AND THE DESIRE TO WANT TO GET BETTER IN PROPER MEAL PLANS.

RENAL/CARDIO/GOUT/DIABETES

LUNCH

OPEN-FACE GRILLED TUNA/CHEESE

SHREDDED CARROT/ROMAINE LETTUCE

FRESH CHERRIES SOUR

4 OUNCES OF BREWED ICE LIME TEA

UNSALTED SEASONINGS

IT IS NOT NECESSARY TO EAT MEAT ALL DAY. GOUT CONDITIONS CAN OCCUR. THIS IS WHERE TOO MUCH CAN BE THE ENEMY. USE EXTRA SHARP CHEESE WITH THE TUNA. TWO TYPES OF PROTEIN BEING SERVED TO BE SURE THE AMOUNT OF PROTEIN YOU USE IS ALLOWED. IF YOU STOP THINKING WHEN EATING THE WORDS (MORE, A LOT, AND STILL HUNGRY WE ALL COULD MAKE IT THROUGH A MEAL SMILE. BE SURE THE CHEESE IS EXTRA SHARP. SWEETEN CHERRIES WITH A SUGAR SUB, SPLIT TOPS, AND SOAK OVERNIGHT. THIS STEP IS FOR THE GOOD OF THE GOUT SIDE.

AS WE GO ALONG WE WILL COME TO THE MEAL PLANNING OF DIABETES AND KIDNEY FAILURE, REMEMBER TO GO BACK TO THE ONES I JUST SHARED IF YOU SHOULD STUMBLE IN YOUR UNDERSTANDING OF CERTAIN AREAS.

BE SURE TO UNDERSTAND WHAT YOU ARE ALLOWED AND WHAT YOU ARE NOT PEANUT BUTTER WAS ONE OF OURS UNTIL THE UNDERSTANDING WAS COMPLETE TO ME. PEANUT BUTTER IS A LEGUME, NOT A NUT, THIS DOES NOT MEAN YOU EAT PEANUTS IN GENERAL, PINE NUTS EITHER, NOT EVEN SOY NUTS. ROBERT CAN BE INCREDIBLY DETERMINED AT TIMES IN WANTING SOMETHING HE CANNOT HAVE LIKE SHELLED PEANUTS, SOY NUTS, JUST A BIG KID. CHECK WITH THE

DIETICIAN OR NUTRITIONIST AT YOUR FACILITY CONCERNING SNACKS.

THERE ARE SNACKS MADE JUST FOR THE RENAL, YOU MUST ASK AND THEN FOLLOW THERE IS NO OTHER WAY. MY HUSBAND IS DIRECTED IN THE WAY HE MUST GO, HE TRIES HARD TO STAY IN HIS OWN LANE. WE TRY EXTREMELY HARD NOT TO EAT OR DO ANYTHING TO DISTRACT HIM FROM HIS HOME RUN. FRIENDS, ALL THAT MUST BE DONE TO MAKE IT TO THIRD BASE IN YOUR STRUGGLE. RUNNING WILL NEVER STOP, SLOWING IT DOWN IS A BLESSING AND GOOD THING. WHEN HE GETS UPSET IN HIS MEAL, ONCE AND A WHILE WE END THE EVENING WITH A GOOD DESSERT, HOMEMADE BREAD PUDDING, SUGAR FREE SHERBET DESSERT, SUGAR FREE JELL O WITH ALLOWED FRUITS WITH VIABLE CHOICE OF WHIP CREAM. CERTAIN FOODS WE KEEP AROUND KNOWING HOW HE IS, IT WORKS OUT WELL. MEAL PLANNING SHOULD NOT CONSIST OF THE SAME FOOD DAY AFTER DAY, I CAN SEE BECOMING UNHAPPY AND BORED. YOU MUST LEARN HOW TO FEEL WHAT YOUR FAMILY MEMBER IS GOING THROUGH EVEN THOUGH YOU ARE NOT, IF THE UNDERSTANDING AND HUMAN AWARENESS IS NOT THERE FROM THE CARETAKER THE BATTLE WILL BE LOST IN TIME SUPPORT IS A MAJOR ISSUE FOR THE RECIPIENT.

WE TRY HARD TO MAKE MEALTIMES A HEALTHY AND HAPPY TIME, IT IS NOT ALWAYS EASY TO DO YOU JUST DO YOUR BEST. I FOUND THAT EATING WHAT AND WHEN ROBERT IS EATING GIVES HIM A BETTER FEELING OF STILL BELONGING TO FAMILIAR FOODS AND A CLOSER FAMILY CONNECTION. YOU CAN TAKE UNFAMILIAR FOODS AND MAKE THEM FAMILIAR, AND

CARING, AND SOME IMAGINATIONS WE DO IT EVERY DAY. YES, FOR SOME PARTS OF THE BODY THAT ARE NOT ABLE TO PRODUCE WHAT IS EXPECTED, LET YOUR MEDICAL STAFF GUIDE YOU TO WELLNESS. YOU MUST MAKE SACRIFICES TO ALLOW THE CHANCE OF REACHING YOUR HEALTH GOAL. YOU ARE RESPONSIBLE FOR 100% OF YOUR MEAL PLANNING.

DEALING WITH FOOD-RELATED CONDITIONS IS NOT A HOP AND A SKIP, IT IS POSSIBLE TO DO IT WELL WITH PROPER GUIDELINES. NO ONE CAN GET WELL PROPERLY WITHOUT ALL OR MOST OF THE NEEDS MET. HOW CAN YOU MAKE A TASTY HOMEMADE CAKE WITHOUT THE PROPER INGREDIENTS? ANY CAKE IS ROBERT'S STAR SMILE.

YES, FRIENDS, I AM TALKING SERIOUSLY, ALL THE WAY. IF YOU ARE NOT SURE YOU ARE ON THE TRACK TO GETTING BETTER, PLEASE TALK TO YOUR MEDICAL TEAM.

IF YOUR MEALS CAN BE MADE HAPPY WITH HEALTHY YOUR CONDITIONS WILL NOT FEEL SO BAD AND CAUSE DEPRESSION. NO ONE SHOULD HAVE TO EAT JUST TO STAY ALIVE, EAT FOR PLEASURE AND FULFILLMENT WITHIN YOU. I FOUND IF THE PERSON UNDERSTANDS WHAT IT IS ALL ABOUT THE CHALLENGE IN GETTING THEM TO ACCEPT THE FOODS MEALS GIVEN HAS A WINNING CHANCE. AS I WRITE ROBERT SITS NEAR AND HE IS MY CENTER OF DIRECTION IN THIS BOOK EVER SO OFTEN I WILL ASK HIM FOR AN OK TO SHARE CERTAIN PAST SITUATIONS HE IN-COUNTERED HIS ANSWER IS ALWAYS" OK." WHAT A GUY.

MANY TIMES, PEOPLE IN GENERAL OLD AND YOUNG CAN BE HARDHEADED, DETERMINE NOT TO CHANGE,

EVERYTHING OFFERED TO HELP THEM THEY TURN BECAUSE EVERYONE GOING THROUGH THIS PART OF THEIR LIFE DOES NOT HAVE ANOTHER'S LOVE, IT SHOULD ALWAYS BE ABOUT DOING IT AS CORRECT AS POSSIBLE UNDER ALL CIRCUMSTANCES. ASK FOR HELP WHEN THE TIME COMES, REMEMBERING THE WORD PRIDE IS JUST THAT A WORD. THERE IS NOT ANY SHAME, WHY? BECAUSE YOU HAVE A PART OF YOUR LIFE THAT YOU NEED HELP AND GUIDANCE. IT IS SO TURNED AROUND SOMETIMES. ALLOW FAMILY AND FRIENDS TO BE THERE FOR YOU, EACH DAY I HAVE LEARNED SOMETHING NEW AND EXCITING ABOUT WHAT I HAVE BEEN SURROUNDED BY ALL MY LIFE, WE ARE NEVER TOO OLD TO OPEN THE DOORS FOR BETTER UNDERSTANDING AND KNOWLEDGE IN MANY AREAS OF LIFE.

MOST STRUGGLES WE HAVE WAS NOT ASKED FOR OR WELCOMED BY US. AT A DOCTOR'S VISIT, A LADY SAT ACROSS FROM ME, AND WE STARTED TALKING. SICKNESSES CAME UP AS USUAL WITH THIS KIND OF ATMOSPHERE. THE THINGS SHE TOLD ME, SHOCKED, AND HURT ME SO BAD, THAT I COULD NOT BELIEVE WHAT I WAS HEARING GENTLY I WAS ABLE TO GET WHO HER PRIMARY DOCTOR WAS. AFTER ONE MONTH OF NOT BEING ABLE TO SHAKE MY FEELINGS ABOUT WHAT I WAS TOLD, I WROTE TO HER DOCTOR TO FIND THE ADDRESS VERY EASILY. I TOLD HIM WHO I WAS, HOW I FELT, AND ALL THE EXTRAS. I DID NOT HEAR FROM HIM FOR QUITE A WHILE, NOW I AM FIGURING OUT WHAT ELSE I CAN DO AND WHAT OTHER STEPS CAN I TAKE? WELL I FINALLY RECEIVED A BEAUTIFUL THOUGHTFUL LETTER FROM HER DOCTOR AND HER FAMILY. THEY HAD NO IDEA THAT THIS HAD BEEN GOING ON. IT WAS INFORMATION NOT FOUND IN BLOOD

TESTS.

I SHARED THIS TO SAY THIS, BE CONCERNED IN FAMILY AND FRIENDS WELFARE NOT JUST YOUR IMMEDIATE FAMILY. YES MANY OF US HAVE OUR DOORS CLOSED VERY TIGHT SO KNOW OTHERS SADNESS, CONCERNS, SICKNESSES, AND FINANCIAL NEEDS, AND ALL THE OTHER HEART SHIPS HAVE A WAY IN. LET ME TELL YOU, IT ALL HAS ITS WAY OF GETTING IN THROUGH THE CRACKS THAT LIFE HAS. MOST OF US BEFORE LIFE IS OVER WILL FEEL SOME KIND OF HARDSHIP AND PAIN. MY SUDDEN FRIEND NEVER KNEW WHAT I DID UNTIL 15 YEARS LATER JUST BEFORE SHE DIED, SHE WAS GLAD I DID, AND IT WAS A BLESSING TO KNOW HER FOR THE BRIEF TIME I DID. IT WAS SOMETHING THAT TOOK PLACE IN MY LIFE AND HERS THAT WAS MEANT TO HAPPEN.

RENAL FAILURE AND DIABETES (2 DIFFERENT HEALTH CONDITIONS). I TRY HARD NOT TO USE THE WORDS DISEASE IT IS SO COLD AND UNCARING. YES, THE DISEASE IS A DISEASE WE WELL KNOW THIS WITHOUT A DOUBT. BOTH ARE DEATH THREATENING BOTH REQUIRE SERIOUS MEAL PLANNING.

(DIABETES AND RENAL) LIKE ANY OTHER COMBINATION MEAL PLAN. EACH NEED MUST BE MET IN MEAL PLANS. IF YOU GRASP THE FOUNDATION OF WHAT IS NEEDED, THIS IS YOUR START, UNDERSTANDING WHAT THE NEEDS ARE AND HOW IMPORTANT. MANY PEOPLE DO NOT HAVE ANYONE TO PREPARE PROPER MEALS OR WHO IS RESPONSIBLE FOR THEIR MEALS. NEEDED ARE THE SKILLS, AND SAD TO SAY, MANY ARE NOT WILLING TO TAKE THE TIME TO LEARN. IF YOU CAN PREPARE YOUR MEAL AND ARE MENTALLY ALERT TO UNDERSTAND, PLEASE USE IT

AND MAKE YOUR FOOD CHOICES CLOSE AS POSSIBLE TO YOUR DIET REGIMEN. I CANNOT GET TO THE STOVE ANYMORE, I THANK GOD I STILL AM ABLE TO SAY WHAT I NEED AND HOW I WANT MY FOOD, TO GIVE ROBERT ALL HE NEEDS IN THE UNDERSTANDING OF HIS NUTRITIONAL NEEDS TO THE BEST OF MY ABILITY, MY CHILDREN ARE RIGHT HERE PURCHASING HIS FOODS PREPPING AND COOKING, WE ARE BLESSED. I AM GENUINELY CONCERNED ABOUT MY FELLOW SENIORS AND THE YOUNG THAT ARE STRUGGLING ALONE TO MEET THEIR IMPORTANT NEEDS. I KNOW IN MY HEART THAT A WHOLE LOT OF PEOPLE CAN MAKE IT THROUGH KNOWING DAILY THAT THEY ARE NOT **ALONE.**

WRITING FROM EXPERIENCE IS A GOOD ROUTE TO FOLLOW, KEEPING IT REAL. MEDICATIONS AND FOOD ARE LIKE A MARRIAGE, BOTH ARE NEEDED TO BECOME WELL AND HAPPY.

 MANY HAVE BEEN MADE TO BELIEVE (DIABETICS) IF THEY TAKE THEIR MEDICATIONS, THEY CAN EAT WHAT YOU WANT AND AS MUCH. WE HAD A FRIEND FIND OUT THE HARD AND SAD WAY. IT ISN'T TRUE SHE LOST HER LIFE IT TOOK A WHILE, BUT IT ALL CAUGHT UP WITH HER BAD EATING WAYS THESE TWO DIETS CAN BE DANGEROUS TO YOUR HEALTH IF NOT FOLLOWED PROPERLY. THE BAD PART CAN SNEAK UP ON YOU.

EATING FOODS FULL OF POTASSIUM, SODIUM, AND PHOSPHORUS IS TASTY, AND FOR MANY OF US TO ENJOY, EVERY FOOD HAS THESE MINERALS FRESH FOODS ARE THE BEGINNING. WE DO NEED THEM TO MAINTAIN OUR BODIES. TOO MUCH OF THEM FOR A KIDNEY PATIENT IS DANGEROUS, THIS IS WHY YOU MUST KEEP UP WITH THE RULES GIVEN. FOODS CAN BLOCK YOUR WAY TO BETTER HEALTH IF NOT PLANNED

PROPERLY, MAKING VARIOUS CONDITIONS WORSE.

YES, WE NEED FRESH FOOD AND OTHER FOODS, BUT NOT BY THE TUB LOADS. REMEMBER WHAT YOUR FIGHT FOR BETTER HEALTH IS ABOUT. OUR BODIES NEED A CERTAIN AMOUNT OF THE ABOVE MINERALS TO FUNCTION HEALTHILY. TOO MUCH IS AS BAD AS TOO LITTLE. THIS IS WHY FOLLOWING YOUR HEALTH TEAM IS IMPORTANT, LET THEM DO THE TELLING, AND WE DO THE LISTENING OK.

MOST HEALTH CONDITIONS ARE ROOTED IN DIET, I STAY AS CLOSE TO THE NUTRITION SIDE AS POSSIBLE. TO DISCUSS ONE WILL BRING IN THE OTHER BECAUSE THEY ARE RELATED IN MANY WAYS, LIKE SEEDS AND DIRT. BOTH ARE NEEDED TO PRODUCE.

IF YOU HAVE KIDNEY FAILURE YOU NEED MEDICAL CARE AND GUIDANCE ALSO IS NEEDED GOOD NUTRITION THE SAME GOES WITH DIABETES.

DO NOT RELY ON UNPROVEN TACTICS, JUST TRY HARD TO DO IT ALL CORRECTLY. YES, WE ALL WITH HEALTH ISSUES WILL SLIP NOW AND THEN, BUT WE CANNOT OUTWEIGH THE REAL. LIFE IS A SHORT STRING THAT GETS SHORTER EVERY MINUTE WE MUST HOLD ON TIGHT NOT TO SLIP AND FALL. EATING IS ONE OF THE MOST EXCITING PLEASURES WE ALL HAVE. TO HAVE IT RESTRICTED IS A HARD PILL TO SWALLOW EVERY DAY. OUR LIVES ARE ALL DIFFERENT, AND SO ARE OUR DESTINIES; DOING OUR BEST IS ALL WE CAN DO. CAN YOU LEAVE THE PROCESSED FOODS YOU ARE SO USED TO ALONE? WHAT ABOUT THE MANY SUGARY FLUIDS YOU USE TO BE ABLE TO DRINK IN ONE DAY? YOU HAVE ALWAYS BEEN ABLE TO EAT THAT BOWL OF CHOCOLATE ICE CREAM, RIGHT? STILL EATING MAC

AND CHEESE, SWEET POTATOES, AND THAT FATTY MEAT SMOTHERED IN DARK LEAFY GREENS? SMILE. FOODS CAN BE MADE HEALTHY.

I WANT ALL OF YOU THAT ARE FIGHTING ALONG WITH MY ROBERT IN THESE CONDITIONS TO USE THIS BOOK TO LEAN ON. READ IT OVER AND OVER, AND REMEMBER IT ALL EVERY TIME YOU BECOME DESPONDENT.

I MENTIONED THAT THE INTAKE OF PROTEIN IN THE EARLY YEARS WAS STRICT. PROTEINS HAD TO BE COUNTED IN EACH MEAL AND MUST ADD UP TO THE AMOUNT ALLOWED FOR THAT DAY. THE THREE AMOUNTS I WAS ASSOCIATED WITH MOST OF THE TIME WERE 40GRAM PRO 60GRAMS,, AND 20 GRAMS .RENAL DIETS.

I WAS RESPONSIBLE FOR THESE MEASUREMENTS TO BE RIGHT ON THE MONEY OR DAMN CLOSE SMILE. WHEN ROBERT BECAME RENAL, I HAD TO RENEW MANY RULES AND SUSTAINED AGAIN THE IMPORTANCE IN THE ILLNESS AND DIET. NOW THE DIET YOU FOLLOW 50 YEARS LATER OFFERS EXCELLENT AMOUNTS OF PROTEIN AND OFFER MORE FAMILIAR FOODS THAT WE ARE ACCUSTOMED TO. CAN YOU NOW IMAGINE HAVING ONLY 20 GRAMS OF PROTEIN TO USE FOR A COMPLETE DAY DEALING WITH 3 MEALS, MEAT ALONE 1 OUNCE. LITTLE MEAT WAS GIVEN BACK THEN, TAKING IT ALL INTO CONSIDERATION IT WAS A JOB IN A JOB IT ALL WAS A LEARNING EXPERIENCE FOR ME, WHAT CAN BE DONE IF IT IS NEEDED. (OVERLOADING IS STILL A NO.)

THE TIME I SPENT IN THIS AREA OF NUTRITION WAS THE BEST. I WILL REPEAT OVER AND OVER FOLLOW YOUR GIVEN DIET CLOSE AND I HAVE FOUND OUT

PRAYER IS A MARVELOUS AND NEEDED ADDITION IN OUR LIVES.

MY STRUCTURE AROUND MY BOOKS WRITTEN IS HAPPY AND HEALTHY IN ANY AGE GROUP. MY BOOKS CAN BE READ BY ALL IT IS MESSAGES THAT CONCERN ALL INCLUDING THIS ONE. DO NOT HESITATE TO PICK UP AND READ BECAUSE YOU SEE THE WORDING SENIOR, REMEMBER YOU WILL BE ONE IN TIME.

WE ALL ARE LIVING IN A WORLD OF MANY SURPRISES, HAPPY ONES, AND SAD ONES. YES, KEEP EYES OPEN TO DIABETES AND KIDNEY DISEASE IT IS ALIVE VERY MUCH SO. WHY DO SO MANY HAVE THIS DISEASE??? LET US PRAY THAT THERE WILL BE LESS AND LESS NEEDED AS THE TIME GOES BY. WE MUST TAKE STEPS TO HELP ONE ANOTHER TODAY AND MAYBE ME TOMORROW. HOW HARD CAN THIS BE, AND YOU ARE BLESSED TO BE ABLE TO FUNCTION WITHOUT STRESS OR HESITATION? THE DOORS ARE OPEN TO TECHNOLOGY EVERY DAY, NEW AND EXCITING THINGS ARE BEING OKAYED FOR THE MANY HEALTH ISSUES THAT ARE FLOATING AROUND ALL OVER THE WORLD. LET US NEVER FORGET TO ALWAYS ADD THE SPIRITUAL NOTES THAT ARE IMPORTANT AND NECESSARY FOR IT ALL TO COME OUT RIGHT.

GETTING BACK TO THE DIETS NEEDED, IN SOME DIETS YOU MUST LEARN HOW TO REMOVE AND REPLACE YOUR FOODS IN ORDER NOT TO INVITE BOREDOM, DIABETES IS ONE. THE HOUSE DIET IS ONE THAT BOTH RENAL AND DIABETICS SHOULD PUSH OVER THE CURB SMILE. IF YOU ARE NOT FAMILIAR WITH THIS TERM, HOUSE DIET YOU NEVER HAVE BEEN IN A HOSPITAL OR CARE FACILITY. THIS DIET IS USUALLY OFFERED TO THOSE WITHOUT SERIOUS OR CONDITIONS THAT THEIR

FOOD INTAKE DOES NOT HAVE TO BE CHANGED. EATING WHAT I WANT AND ALL I WANT SEEMS TO BE STUBBORN MARK IN MANY, OR SOMEONE WILL SAY MY MOM OR GRANNY DID IT THEY HAD NO PROBLEMS, IF YOU ARE FROM MY GENERATION STARTING WITH THE 1940'S IF THERE WAS SOMETHING GOING ON IT WAS NOT DISCUSSED AROUND US IF MY GRANNY OR PARENTS HAD HEALTH ISSUES I DID NOT KNOW TO WHAT EXTENT. MANY WAYS AND RULES PARENTS HAVE NOW HAD NO COMPARISON IN MY TIME. DEATH OF A LOVE ONE TOLD THEIR STORY OF THEIR LIFE.

OBESITY IS A HARD STONE TO MOVE FROM OUR LIVES, WE JUST MUST DO OUR BEST TO BRING TO THE MARK IT NEEDS TO BE. AND BELIEVE ME IT IS NOT EASY NOT ONE BIT. DO NOT LET THE WORLD DECIDE FOR YOU, DO IT FOR YOU. DO NOT KEEP A HIDDEN LOCK ON YOUR HEALTH AND NEVER BE ASHAMED IF YOU ARE REACHING OUT FOR HELP AND TRYING HARD TO FOLLOW THROUGH. WE FEEL GOOD ROBERT AND I TO SHARE WE NEVER KNOW WHO AND WHERE SOMEONE MAY BE MOTIVATING IN TAKING GOOD CHARGE IN THEIR LIVES FROM WHAT IS BEING SHARED. KEEPING A LOCK AND KEY ON OUR HEALTH CONDITIONS WILL NOT MAKE THEM GET BETTER OR DISAPPEAR. SHARING IS A GOOD AND SOLID STEP IN HELPING HUMANITY, NEVER LET $$$$$ BE A GUIDE TRY YOUR HEART. WE AS A FAMILY ARE PROUD THAT ROBERT AGREED TO DISCUSS THE LANDMARKS OF HIS CONDITION. I HAVE HEARD SOME SAY" HOW CAN SHE OR HE TALK PERSONAL HEALTH TO THE WORLD"? THIS IS HOW MORE HEALING AND SOLID INFORMATION IS GIVEN TO SOMEONE FOR THEY CAN DO SOMETHING WITH IT. IF THE SCIENTISTS FELT THIS WAY, WE WOULD ALL BE A DYING BUNCH.

CONTINUE TO STAY WITH ME; WE WILL GET SOME
RECIPES FOR THE RENAL DIET AND DIABETIC. YOU
NEED THE NECESSARY INFORMATION BEFORE I GET
STARTED.

THERE ARE FOODS AND MINERALS THAT WE DO NOT
USE BECAUSE ALTHOUGH THEY ARE OK FOR DIABETICS
BUT NOT FOR THE RENAL. SUCH AS POTASSIUM,
SODIUM, SALT AND PHOSPHOROUS THIS IS ALERTNESS
FOR THE RENAL EATER. PRACTICE USING FRESH
FOODS AND PRODUCES TO CREATE TASTY RECIPES.
THE FACT THAT IT HAS BEEN PROVEN THAT FRESH IS
BEST, THIS DOES NOT MEAN THAT NONE OF THE ABOVE
MINERALS ARE NOT THERE, THEY ARE AND IN THEIR
STRONGEST ADDITIONS. I DO KNOW I HAVE SAID THIS
MORE THAN ONCE, BELIEVE ME REPEATING IS MUCH
NECESSARY. WE READ A COUPLE PAGES BACK, AND
YOU HAVE FORGOTTEN, SOME OF WHAT YOU READ
REAL QUICK MOST OF US DO THIS AT MY AGE, SO WHAT
NOT ONLY OLDER YEARS DOES THIS ALSO THE YOUNG
HAS THEIR DAYS ALSO SMILE. KEEPING THE FOODS
AND MINERALS AS THEY HAVE BEEN DIRECTED TO YOU
IS THE WAY WE GO. I FIND IT SAFE TO JUST FOLLOW
THE RULES OF THE DIET WHEN YOU GO PASS THE
RULES AND MAKE YOUR OWN WRONG ONES, ALL THE
SUFFERING AND DISMAY FALLS ON YOU.

TO GET IT ALL RIGHT 100% WILL NOT BE EASY, WE
WILL CONTINUE TO TRY OUR BEST. FRIENDS AND
FAMILY ENJOY HELPING SO YOU MUST HANDLE HOW
THE FOODS HE SHOULD EAT ARE ADDRESSED
CAREFULLY, INCLUDING THEIRS. WE MISTAKE SODIUM
WITH SALT, THEY ARE NOT THE SAME IN A FEW WAYS.
ALTHOUGH SALT IS TAKEN FROM THE MINERAL
SODIUM, IODINE IS ADDED SO WE CAN USE IT IN OUR

FOODS. FOODS ARE OFTEN GIVEN TO ROBERT AS A GIFT OR SERVED AT ANOTHER'S HOME, THEY WILL SAY "THIS IS OK IT IS NO SALT" WE REJECT IT BECAUSE I KNOW THE PRODUCT IS LOADED WITH SODIUM. THIS MINERAL CAN BE FOUND IN ABOUT ANYTHING IF YOU DO NOT READ INGREDIENT LABELS WITH THE UNDERSTANDING IN WHAT YOU NEED TO KNOW, YOU CAN NEVER BE SURE OF THE ROUTE YOU ARE TAKING IS RIGHT. SO WHEN YOU READ SODIUM INVOLVED IN ANY INGREDIENT LABEL BEWARE. FLUID RESTRICTION COMES WITH KIDNEY CONDITIONS SO WHEN YOU DECIDE WHAT DRINKS WILL HAVE EACH DAY I ALWAYS INCLUDE WATER FOR PART OF ROBERTS.

RENAL MEAL PLANNING CAN BE A WINNER. ANY CONDITION RELATED TO FOODS CAN BE HAPPY. BAKE YOUR OWN CAKES AND OTHER DESSERTS IF NEEDED, BISCUITS, ALL THOSE FAMILIAR GOODIES. I MENTIONED EARLIER NO PROCESSED FOODS. WE HAVE BREAD PUDDING, CORN STARCH VANILLA PUDDINGS, EGGNOG RICE PUDDINGS, FRUITED JELLO USING PROPER FRUITS, AND MANY OTHER DESSERTS. LEAFY GREEN VEGETABLES ARE OUT; BEETS AND CUCUMBERS ARE HIS FAVORITES. ALSO, ARE GONE FROM HIS DIET. HE NOW ENJOYS FRENCH GREEN BEANS, WHITE CABBAGE, CAULIFLOWER, CANDY CARROTS USING SUGAR SUB, EGGPLANT, AND OTHERS, BEING AWARE OF HOW OFTEN AND HOW MUCH.

YOU KNOW FROZEN FOODS HAVE COME AN EXCEPTIONALLY LONG WAY THROUGH THE YEARS BUT KEEP YOUR EYES OPEN TO THE AMOUNTS OF SODIUM INTAKE. I AM POSITIVE YOU HAVE A CHART TO FOLLOW, PLEASE PRACTICE USING IT FOR EVERY FOOD SO THAT ALL THE FOODS MENTIONED CAN BE MADE HEALTHY

SO BOTH SIDES CAN ENJOY THEM.

SOY MIGHT JUST GIVE YOU WHAT YOU ARE LOOKING FOR. DOUBLE-CHECK THIS FIRST WE USE SOME OF THE MILK BUT NOT THE BEANS. YES, I KNOW SOY PRODUCTS ARE MADE FROM BEANS. WE USE NON-DAIRY PRODUCTS. BE CAREFUL WITH YOUR MELON AREAS, SUCH AS CANTALOUPE, CRENSHAW MELON, OTHER MELONS, PRUNES, FIGS, DATES, RAISINS, NECTARINES, ORANGES, MANGO, AND PAPAYA. SORRY YOU CANNOT HAVE IT SMILE. I STICK TO THE FRUITS HE CAN HAVE WITHOUT OVERLOADING ON THEM, REMEMBERING THE DIABETIC SIDE. A FIG HERE AND THERE OCCASIONALLY, ALONG WITH ANOTHER ALLOWED FRUIT, WORKS OUT WELL I AM TALKING ABOUT ONE FIG, NOT FOUR. CHILLED WATERMELON AND BERRIES, FRESH SLICED BAKED APPLE AND PEARS, STRAWBERRY SHORTCAKE MADE WITH HOMEMADE POUND CAKE, AND SLICED FRESH STRAWBERRIES. THIS IS HOW I DO IT. FOR THE POTATOES, I DO A SOAK AND ALLOW THE HAPPY TO EAT TWICE A WEEK AT THE MOST. YES, THIS IS AN IMPORTANT DIET; FIND A PLACE FOR HAPPINESS MUCH AS PORTION CONTROL AND   EATING THE SAME FOODS TOO OFTEN IS A POOR ROUTINE, USE A VARIETY OF FOODS AND MEAL PLANS.

IF YOU ARE FOLLOWING A RENAL DIET, I AM POSITIVE YOU HAVE THE EATING OUTLINES.

I WILL NOW GO TO THE DIABETIC RULES IN EATING. LATER YOU WILL CAREFULLY BE SHOWN HOW TO TAKE THESE TWO IMPORTANT DIETS CONNECTING THEM TO EACH OTHER IN RECIPES AND, MOST OF ALL, DAILY MEAL PLANNING, THERE WILL BE LOW CHOLESTEROL AND FAT ALLOWANCES ALSO I WILL BE USING

ROBERT'S DIETS AND A FEW OF OTHERS THAT MIGHT HAVE MORE THAN ROB HAS, TAKE SOME OF MINE BUT CHECK WITH YOUR DOCTOR FIRST. I AM NOT DRAFTING THIS BOOK TO SHOW ALL MISTAKES OR FAULTS BUT TO LET YOU READ HOW YOU CAN ADJUST TO YOUR NEW WAY OF EATING WITHOUT BITTERNESS OR CONFUSION. NEVER FEEL YOU ARE ALONE. WE LIVE IN DIFFERENT COUNTRIES AND CITIES AROUND THE GLOBE, BUT IN IT ALL, WE UNITE IF NOTHING BUT WITH OUR ILLNESSES AND HOPES. PEOPLE JUST WILL NOT ADMIT THEIR STRUGGLES, WHICH IS THEIR RIGHT, BUT MANY TIMES CAN BE FOOLISH. THERE IS HELP FOR YOU SOMEWHERE ONCE WE OWN UP TO OUR HEALTH ISSUES, OUR PATHWAYS WILL NOT BE SO HARD TO FOLLOW. PATIENCE AND TIME ARE NEEDED FOR THIS CHANGE LIFE HAS DROPPED IN OUR ARMS; TO CONTINUE LIFE, WE MUST DO WHAT WE MUST DO. FAMILIES ARE GOING THROUGH GRAVE CHANGES IN THEIR LIVES; SOMETHING NEW IS BEING ADDED EVERY SECOND. NEVER TAKE ON YOUR OWN ANYTHING CONCERNING THE WELFARE OF YOUR HEALTH WITHOUT A PROFESSIONAL IN THAT AREA OF HEALTH PERMISSION TO PROCEED OR REJECT.

IF YOU ARE A CARETAKER AND CONFUSED IN NUTRITION, ASK FOR HELP AND MORE GUIDANCE. NEVER HESITATE; STAY ON THE CORRECT TRACK IN WHAT YOU ARE DOING WHEN YOU ARE CARING FOR ANOTHER THEIR WELL-BEING IS IN YOUR HANDS. THEY WILL GIVE YOU A RUN FOR YOUR MONEY, MOST OF US WILL WHEN IT COMES TO OUR LIKES AND DISLIKES, IN OUR FOODS, IF THIS KIND OF ATTITUDE WERE SHOWN IN DOING IT RIGHT NOT WRONG THE NUMBER OF SICKNESSES WOULD BE CUT IN HALF.

DIABETES IS, LIKE MANY OTHER HEALTH CONDITIONS, BEEN AROUND FOR QUITE A WHILE AND GROWING. MANY HAVE DENIAL BELIEVING THE PANCREAS IS NOT ABLE TO DO THE JOB AS WELL ANYMORE OR AT ALL, THIS CONDITION MAKES THE BODY SENSITIVE TO UN-PROPER CARE. DOES DIABETES COME FROM EATING TOO MANY SWEETS, OR I WILL SAY SUGAR? NO, THERE ARE PARTNERS IN THIS CONDITION. I GIVE IT THE UN-BALANCE OF EATING FOR MOST OF THE 3 NUTRIENTS, FATS, CARBOHYDRATES, AND PROTEINS TOO MUCH OF ONE OR TWO AND NOT ENOUGH OF THE OTHER OR OTHERS., YES IT CAN BE INHERITED AND OTHER WAYS ALSO, THE IMPORTANCE OF IT ALL IS TO EAT AS HEALTHY AS POSSIBLE CHOOSING GOOD NUTRITION. YOU MAY NOT BE EATING PLENTY OF SIMPLE SUGAR (CANDY, HEAVILY SUGARED FOODS, AND SNACKS); WHAT ABOUT THE COMPLEX SUGARS (PIES, CAKES, BREAD, PASTA, ETC. THESE FOODS CARRY THEIR OWN STYLE OF SUGAR ALL THE BLOOD KNOWS THAT HERE COMES SOME SUGAR. KEEP UP WITH YOUR BLOOD WORK, FOLLOW YOUR CALORIES ALLOWED GIVEN FOR EACH DAY, PLAN YOUR MEALS, TO MAKE SURE YOUR PORTIONS ARE CORRECT, AND LEARN AS MUCH INFORMATION ON EATING WITH DIABETES. IF SNACKS ARE CALCULATED FOR YOU EACH MEAL, BE SURE TO HAVE THEM AND REMEMBER YOUR SNACKS ARE A PART OF YOUR ORIGINAL AMOUNT OF CALORIES EAT THEM. AGAIN, YOUR MEDICAL STAFF AND DIETICIAN OR NUTRITIONIST ARE YOUR LEADERS IN THIS AREA. STOP FALLING IN LOVE WITH JUST CERTAIN FOODS BETTER THAN OTHERS MOST OF US DO, WE MUST EAT A VARIETY EACH HAS ITS OWN SPECIAL NUTRITION DNA. ARE THE RULES FOR DIABETES SIMPLE? OVERLOADING IS A NO. IN BETWEEN MEALS SNACKING, UNLESS IT IS YOUR SNACK, YOU SHOULD HAVE TIME FOR YOUR

MORNING, AFTERNOON, AND EVENING STACK, DO NOT
SNACK WHEN YOU GET READY TO FOLLOW THE DIET.

BEWARE OF THE KIND OF SNACKS YOU CHOOSE.
ALWAYS HAVE AN IDEA WHAT YOUR GLUCOSE IS IN
CASE YOU ARE ASKED. STOP TRIPLING UP ON MEALS
THAT YOU DID NOT EAT WHEN YOU SHOULD HAVE, AND
DO NOT PUT LUNCH AND DINNER MEALS TOGETHER OR
BREAKFAST AND NOONTIME SNACKS UNLESS YOU
HAVE BEEN TOLD BY YOUR MEDICAL STAFF. YOUR
MEAL PLANNING AND EATING HABITS ARE IMPORTANT.
THESE ARE IMPORTANT BECAUSE YOU NEED BALANCE
IN THIS DIET, YOU WILL HAVE BETTER GLUCOSE
READINGS

YOU DO NOT WANT AN EXTREMELY LOW READING AT
LUNCH AND SKY-HIGH AT DINNER. WE READ OUR
GLUCOSE ABOUT 3 TIMES A DAY, I WAS ASKING FOR
STRIPS LIKE CRAZY FOR ME WHEN I FIRST BECAME A
DIABETIC, LEARNING HOW MY MEALS AFFECTED MY
SUGAR. MOST OF ALL, STOP FOLLOWING FRIENDS,
FAMILY MEMBERS AND NEW ACQUAINTANCES IN THEIR
MEAL PLANNING FOLLOW YOUR DIET REGIMENT.

THESE DESSERTS HAVE PROVEN TO BE GOOD FOR
ROBERT, HIS REPORT CARD TELLS HIM THAT.

DIABETES AND HIGH BLOOD PRESSURE ARE THE
NUMBER ONE CONDITIONS IN HAVING KIDNEY FAILURE.
THERE IS MUCH MORE GOING ON, BUT THESE TWO ARE
MY INTERESTS BECAUSE I AM IN THE ZONE.

THERE IS A LEVEL, LIKE ANYTHING ELSE, OUR BODIES
MUST MAINTAIN FOR ALL ORGANS AND CELLS CAN BE
ON THE SAME LINE. THIS IS WHY DOCTOR VISITS AND
BLOOD WORK IS ESSENTIAL. OUR BLOOD TELLS THE

STORY OF WHAT IS GOING ON INSIDE THE BODY. WE OURSELVES CAN SEE WE HAVE A RASH IT DOES NOT WORK IN AREAS WE CANNOT SEE.

MY LOVED ONE IS GOING THROUGH THIS TIME NOW, AND FOR A WHILE, I TRY TO SUPPORT HIM IN HIS MEALS AND MENTAL ACCEPTANCE. WITH A GOOD LEADER, HIS DOCTOR MAKES ALL RUN AS SMOOTHLY AS POSSIBLE. THANKS, DOCTOR BRENDA HOFFMAN. IT IS ALL ABOUT CARING FOR AND SHARING WITH ANY ILLNESS.

EATING PROPERLY IS IMPORTANT IN MANY WAYS FOR THE RENAL. THE FOLLOWING INFORMATION GIVEN CONCERNING YOUR ALLOWANCE IS ESSENTIAL DAILY.

THERE ARE MANY SERIOUS HEALTH CONDITIONS KIDNEY DISEASE IS AT THE TOP OF THE LIST FOR ME NOT ONLY TO BE CONNECTED TO MY HUSBAND BUT THE YEARS WORKING WITH PATIENTS LIKE MANY OF US WHO ARE SET IN WAYS OF EATING THAT IS HARD TO CHANGE. BEING ON A THIN LINE OF BEING WELCOMED MYSELF I WANTED AND HAD TO SHARE ALL THAT I KNOW CONCERNING EATING WITH RENAL FAILURE. NOTHING IS EASY WHEN IT IS NECESSARY FOR US TO DO IT. HAVING OTHER CONDITIONS ONLY MAKES THE BATTLE A HARDER FIGHT.

THERE ARE TWO MAJOR CONCERNS IN THE MEAL PLANNING OF A RENAL DIET. PHOSPHORUS AND POTASSIUM ARE THE ENEMIES, WHY" BECAUSE THEY OFFER MINERALS THAT THE KIDNEY CANNOT HANDLE, SIM PLEA AS THAT STICKING TO THE TRITON SIDE. I AM HERE TO SHARE ONLY THAT AREA MY QUALIFICATION DOES NOT GO ANYWHERE NEAR THE MEDICAL AREA OF ANY DISEASES. I WANT TO BE CLEAR WITH KNOWN

MISUNDERSTANDINGS TO MY READERS. I WILL GO OVER THE BASIC STYLE OF EATING THAT GOES ON IN MY HOME, SOME RECIPES THAT MY HUSBAND HAS FOUND TASTY AND GOOD CHANGES IN CERTAIN DAILY STYLES.

I MENTIONED EARLIER THAT THE DIETS THAT RENAL PATIENTS HAD TO FOLLOW 50 YEARS AGO WERE VERY RIGID. TODAY, THE MEAL PLANNING AND ACCEPTABLE FOODS OFFERED ARE AWESOME. TAKE TO HEART WHAT YOUR LEADERS ARE OFFERING AND WORK WITH IT WITH ALL YOU MUST GIVE. WE ARE THE PATIENTS WHO MAKE IT ALL RIGHT FOR YOU. THERE ARE MANY AROUND THE WORLD THAT ARE SUFFERING AND SEE NO WAY OUT, MANY YOUNG INCLUDED. IT IS SAD AND HEARTBREAKING WHEN YOU HAVE PEOPLE THAT CAN RECEIVE HELP, GUIDANCE, AND OPEN INFORMATION FOR THEIR WELLNESS AND WILL NOT EVEN TRY. REMEMBER, LIFE OWES US NOTHING WE OWE LIFE BECAUSE WE ARE STILL LIVING.

I HAD A FRIEND SOME TIME AGO CALL ME; SHE HAD JUST STARTED EATING A RENAL DIET. THIS DAY WAS A SURPRISE FOR ME. I WAS FEELING A LITTLE DOWN AND HAD BEEN THINKING OF HER AND HER FAMILY FOR A COUPLE OF DAYS, BUT I HAD MISPLACED MY PERSONAL PHONE BOOK AND HAD BEEN TOO LAZY TO FILE IT ON THE COMPUTER JUST IN CASE SOMETHING LIKE THIS HAPPENED. SHE HAD BEEN ILL FOR A WHILE; I WOULD NOT HAVE KNOWN IF I HAD NOT CALLED HER. THIS IS WHAT OLD AND DEAR FRIENDS DO. SHE DISCUSSED HER ILLNESS, AND I, IN RETURN, DISCUSSED HUBBIES AND MINE. AFTER SHE FINISHED, QUESTIONED HER WHO TOLD HER TO EAT THE STYLE DIET SHE WAS EATING. TO MAKE THE STORY SHORT,

SHE DECIDED TO FOLLOW HER OWN AND HER SISTERS.

THE FOLLOWING IS WHAT SHE HAS BEEN EATING. I AM PRAYING THAT AFTER TALKING TO HER, SHE HAS STOPPED.

IN THE LAST WEEK, SHE HAS HAD TOMATO SALADS, ASSORTED MELON, AND CREAMY COTTAGE CHEESE.

POTATO SALAD MADE WITHOUT SOAKING THE POTATOES, PEANUT BUTTER JELLY SANDWICH AT LUNCH, SWEET POTATO

PIE, ORANGE JUICE, THE FOOD GOES ON AND ON SHE IS ON THE RIGHT TRACK NOW BECAUSE I TOLD HER SOME.

AND REAL HORRORS CONCERNING WHAT SHE IS DOING. I TOOK THE SUBJECT THAT WAS MAKING HER CONDITION WORSE I FEEL AND PRAY. THE SONG SAYS IT ALL THAT IS *WHAT FRIENDS ARE FOR!*

LUNCH

UNSALTED CARROT/CAULIFLOWER SOUP

EGG SALAD SANDWICH ON WHITE BREAD

SMALL APPLE

SMALL TEA

SIMPLE BUT HEALTHY.

DINNER

Baked chicken /no skin

Buttered rice/parsley

Green French beans

Small Cabbage slaw

Small, sliced strawberries and blueberries.

Cook green beans in unsalted chicken stock. Mix a small amount of light mayonnaise in the slaw.

Two simple tasty meals following amounts and how often.

Stay away from foods given, such as

Oranges lemons

Cantaloupe/Honeydew

Raisins, figs, dates

Sweet potatoes

White potatoes if not prepped properly.

The list goes on and on in both areas of allowances.

Our Desserts for Renal

1. Strawberry rice pudding.

2. Homemade slice pound cake/top with fruit

3. Baby berry cobbler/shortbread cookies

4. Unsalted rice cakes/cream cheese/grape preserves

5. Shortbread cookies/cornstarch vanilla pudding

6. Mix can fruit in juice, not syrup/sugar-free jell o

7. Homemade bread pudding/FLAVORED with banana and pecan. (Not the fruit or nut)

**Allowed flavoring can be a plus.

8. Fresh sweet cherries

9. Sherbet float (using diet 7-up)

10. Frozen grapes/can pears.

Yes, rejection of food choices does appear when the patient is not involved in the choices. Keep the receiver of meals always involved.

The desserts shown are only a part of the recipes. Baby food is a step we found to be helpful in making sauces, desserts and also smoothies.

IMPORTANT) READ LABELS ON FOODS PURCHASED, THIS WILL SAVE YOU DISAPPOINTMENTS AND GIVE BETTER UNDERSTANDINGS IN YOUR NEEDS.

WE PURCHASED AN ITEM ONCE AND WERE PLEASED, SHOPPING FAST, SMILED WHEN READY TO PREP DINNER FOUND THE POTASSIUM WAS SKY HIGH THIS DOES HAPPEN, BE AWARE WHEN PREPPING MEALS DOUBLE CHECK.

DESSERTS FOR DIABETICS (SUGAR-FREE)

1. FRESH FRUITS (MOST)
2. PUDDINGS
3. PINEAPPLE CHEESECAKE
4. BERRY SHORTCAKE
5. FROZEN YOGURTS
6. CHUTNEY
7. SHORTBREAD COOKIES (4)
8. JELL O
9. FIG/APRICOT COMPOTE

10 PEANUT BUTTER SURPRISE *

THE ABOVE IS THE VARIETY OF CHOICES WE MUST USE WHAT WE CAN.

DO NOT BE ALARMED ABOUT THIS CHEESECAKE. IT IS PUT TOGETHER USING ALL THE GIVEN RULES AND THE SHORTCAKE. RENAL CAN HAVE THE BERRY CAKE (THE BERRIES MUST BE EATEN AT A LOW. AS I

EXPLAINED EARLIER, EVEN FRUIT AND VEGGIES MUST BE ACCOUNTED FOR AND EATEN AS DESCRIBED AT A LOW.

I WILL NOW SHARE WITH YOU AS CLEARLY AS POSSIBLE TO CREATE A MEAL (BOTH DIETS PROPERLY). READ SOLID INFORMATION ON HOW OTHER HEALTH-RELATED CONDITIONS AND MEAL PLANNING CAN CONNECT LIKE A PUZZLE; ALL IT TAKES IS THE WORD (HOW) EXPLAINED AND SHARED WITH YOU. WE ARE THE SENIOR HOOD STRUGGLING TO STAY HEALTHY AND HAPPY) ALSO THE YOUNG GENERATION BY USING PREVENTIVE HEALTH PROCEDURES.

RENAL/DIABETIC/LOW CHOL(CHOL.-CHOLESTEROL)

*32 OUNCES OF FLUIDS ALLOWED WITHIN 24 HOURS.

LUNCH

4 OUNCES VEGGIE BROTH

2 OZ. LEAN PORK LOIN

2 SLICES WHITE BREAD

SHREDDED LETTUCE HEARTS

RED SLICE ONIONS

1 TBSP LIGHT MAYONNAISE

1 SMALL FRESH APPLE

4-OUNCE CHILLED WATER

SNACK TIME

2 GRAHAM CRACKER SQUARES/4 OUNCES EGG SHAKE.

ONE EGG/VAN FLAVOR/CINNAMON/NON-DAIRY MILK, SUGAR SUB. BLEND WELL

**12 OUNCES OF FLUIDS USED. **

DIABETIC SIDE	RENAL SIDE
SOUP- OK	ACCEPTABLE
MEAT-OK	ACCEPT
VEGGIES OK	ACCEPT
BREAD-OK	ACCEPT
DESSERT-OK	ACCEPT
BEVERAGE OK	ACCEPT

I HOPE THIS OUTLINE SHOWS YOU A LITTLE MORE CLEARLY HOW WE DO IT.

THE REST OF THE DAY, NOT EXCEEDING 32 OUNCES, TRY HARD TO STAY IN THE PROPER CIRCLE OF ALLOWANCE. IT CAN BE ROUGH ON HOT DRY DAYS. HAVING HOMEMADE ICED FRUIT CUPS AROUND HELPS. WE USE 4-OUNCE CUPS. ALLOWING ROBERT 4 DURING THE DAY ALLOWS ME TO WORK THE OTHER 16 OUNCES TO BE USED FOR THE REMAINING OF THE DAY.

You will observe that as I go along this hard but fair road of health, some humor will be added, and I feel needed. This is not a sad story I am sharing life as it is in our lives. I am a member of other conditions, and they are not easy to receive either. We try hard to eat happily and healthily in our home, it can be trying at times. I feel that no matter what diet regimen you must follow, happiness can be fitted in some way. Food is a major part of living.

The flavor is what most of us want.

A RENAL MEAL

BREAKFAST

Peaches/pears

½ cup OATMEAL

2 EGGS made over light.

½ plain BAGEL /jelly/CREAM CHEESE

MARGARINE

Sugar Substitute

4 ounces NON-DAIRY MILK

+ 4 ounces WATER

+ 4 ounces cup hot beverage

= 12 ounces of fluids used. **

LUNCH

½ CUP SOUP 4 OUNCES

LEAN BURGER/ROLL/BABY SPINACH

COOKED ONIONS

LIGHT MAYONNAISE

APPLESAUCE

4 OUNCES BREWED ICE COFFEE

ICE 4 OUNCES

12 OUNCES OF FLUID USED.

DINNER

STEAMED SCALLOPS/RICE/CARROTS.

SEASONED FRENCH GREEN BEANS

MARGARINE

SHORTBREAD COOKIE DESSERT

4 OUNCES PINEAPPLE JUICE

4 OUNCES OF CHILLED WATER

8 OUNCES OF FLUID WERE USED.

**ALL FLUIDS INTAKE OF 32 OUNCES USED WITHIN 3 MEALS. **

THIS IS JUST AN EXAMPLE OF HOW IT CAN BE DONE WITHOUT YOU GETTING TURNED ALL AROUND. BE SURE YOU USE THE PROPER CONDIMENTS AND FATS. DO IT YOUR WAY, JUST BE SURE IT IS THE CORRECT WAY.

IN GOOD TIME YOU WILL FIND YOUR OWN WAYS TO GET THE PROPER FLUIDS IN YOUR DAILY MEALS AND BE ABLE TO STAY IN YOUR PROPER COUNT. WE MAKE MILK A PART OF THE DAY'S MEALS, ALSO WATER; NOT ALL THREE FIT IN SOME ARE ALLOWED A HARD CANDY IN BETWEEN MEALS, BUT THIS IS UP TO YOUR DIRECTOR (ROBERT IS NOT).

STAY AWAY FROM CANNED AND PACKAGED SOUPS, MOST ARE FILLED WITH HIGH SODIUM, SALT, AND OTHER MINERALS YOU DO NOT NEED EXTRAS IN YOUR MEALS.

STAY ALERT. IF A LABEL DOES NOT SAY THE WORD SALT, THIS DOES NOT MEAN THE SAME ENEMY IS NOT INCLUDED. I HAVE FOUND THIS PART OF IT ALL VERY CONFUSING FOR MANY, RESTRICTED FROM THIS MINERAL. THERE ARE OTHER TERMS USED THAT MEAN SODIUM.

THE HARDEST ISSUE FOR ROBERT IS PORTION CONTROL. BEING A MAN THAT HAS HAD A GREAT APPETITE ALL HIS LIFE, THIS IS EXPECTED OF HIM. UNDERSTANDING AND SACRIFICING ARE THE TOOLS THAT MUST BE USED BY PATIENTS AND CARETAKERS. THERE HAVE BEEN MANY TIMES I WANTED FOOD AND

CHANGED AND ENJOYED WHAT I WAS TRYING HARD FOR HIM TO ENJOY. PUTTING YOURSELF IN THE OTHER PERSON'S SHOES NEEDS TO BE DONE MORE OFTEN. EVEN WHEN THEY ARE DOING WELL WITH THEIR DIET. IT MAKES YOU THE SUPPORTER, STRONGER AND MORE UNDERSTANDING.

I AM GOING INTO A DIABETIC DIET. THIS CONDITION, IF NOT FOLLOWED WITH ALL BASES COVERED MEDICALLY AND NUTRITIONALLY, CAN BE HARMFUL TO YOUR HEALTH. THIS DIET ALSO HAS NO AGE LIMIT. THERE ARE ASSORTED REASONS FOR IT, BUT I WILL LEAVE THAT UP TO THE MEDICAL WORLD. FOLLOWING YOUR DIET AND MEDICATIONS. FOOD IS ONE OF THE KEYS TO DIABETES. THIS IS A DIET THAT SHOULD NOT BE TAKEN LIGHTLY, THE SAME AS THE RENAL DIET. DIABETICS CAN EAT HAPPILY AND HEALTHILY MOST OF THE TIME WHEN FOLLOWING THE CORRECT DIET REGIMEN. READ FOOD PACKAGES AND BOTTLE LABELING; NOT JUST THE NUTRITIONAL FACTS AND INGREDIENTS ARE IMPORTANT ALSO. THIS IS NECESSARY TO HAVE A BETTER UNDERSTANDING AND KEEP ON THE RIGHT LINES IN YOUR NUTRITIONAL HEALTH NEEDS.

THE MEAL PLANS A DIABETIC FOLLOWED BEFORE THE CONDITION CAN EASILY BE TURNED INTO A NEW MEAL PLAN. I AM TALKING ONLY ABOUT THE AVERAGE EVERYDAY FAMILIAR FOODS, NOT THE ADDITIONS OR THE WORSE WAYS. I WILL SHARE AN EXAMPLE OF HOW I DO IT.

ROBERT HAS ALWAYS BEEN ABLE TO ENJOY THE FOLLOWING FOODS FOR MANY YEARS.

PIES, CAKES, CREAM SANDWICH COOKIES, POTATO CHIPS, PRETZELS, FRENCH FRIES, POTATOES, SEASONED GREENS WITH SALTY MEATS, RICE WITH HEAVY GRAVIES, MACARONI AND CHEESE, AND MOST MEATS.

THIS IS HOW IT CAN STILL BE THERE BUT IN A HEALTHIER WAY.

PIE

SLICE OR DICE FRESH FRUITS, ALLOWED, AND ADD A CORNSTARCH THICKENING PLUS SUGAR SUBSTITUTE AND FLAVORING. LET COOK UNTIL THICKEN. MAKE A HOMEMADE CRUST (USE GRAHAM CRACKERS OR UNSALTED PLAIN CRACKERS) IT CAN BE DONE IN SIMPLE, QUICK WAYS,

SANDWICH COOKIES

SUGARED CREAM FILLINGS-SHORT BREAD COOKIE CENTER WITH LOW SUGAR, LOW FAT THICKEN THE PUDDING.

POTATO CHIPS

TRY USING VEGGIES LIKE TARO ROOT OR PLANTAINS. NO SALT OR ADDED SUGARS. CHIPS COOKED IN UNSATURATED OIL, TRYING SOMETHING NEW WILL NOT HURT. TRY YOUR HEALTH STORES.

FRENCH FRIES

TRY OVEN FRIES, OR PURCHASE A CRISPY SHEET

OR AIR FRYER, THEY SELL VEGGIE FRIES, TOO. MADE WITH CAULIFLOWER AND ZUCCHINI.

COOK GREENS IN VEGGIE, CHICKEN, LOW-FAT, AND SODIUM BROTH OR STOCK. CHECK OUT LIQUID SMOKE, AND READ IF IT IS GOOD FOR YOU IF YOU WANT THAT SMOKED TASTE.

MAC/CHEESE-

USE HEALTHY MARGARINE, LOW-FAT CHOLESTEROL, SODIUM CHEESES, AND LOW-FAT MILK. STOP OVERLOADING ON FOOD, A SERVING IS JUST WHAT IT IS. IT DOES NOT TAKE ENORMOUS AMOUNTS OF CHEESE TO HAVE A SATISFYING MACARONI AND CHEESE CASSEROLE. REPLACE PASTA WITH CAULIFLOWER.

THE ABOVE IS JUST A QUICK GUIDELINE THAT CAN BE USED IN TURNING YOUR MEAL PLANNING AROUND AND STAYING CONNECTED WITH FAMILIAR FOODS. PORTION CONTROL WE HAVE FOUND FOR ROBERT HAS BEEN THE HARDEST CHANGE, WE KNOW IT IS ONE OF THE MOST IMPORTANT STEPS HE HAS TO BE ABLE TO CLIMB IN HIS DIET. (SO FAR, SO GOOD).

ATTENTION!!!!

NEVER BE ASHAMED OF WHAT FOODS YOU PURCHASE. IF YOU HAVE A NEED FOR BABY FOOD, YOU PURCHASE IT PROUDLY. WHATEVER IS DONE CONCERNING YOUR HEALTH NEEDS IS YOURS.

KEEP THE TWO DIETS SEPARATE BUT YET CONNECTED IN FOOD NEEDS

PLEASE FOLLOW EACH DIET AND

CONDITION WITHIN ITSELF. A BETTER UNDERSTANDING CAN DEVELOP WHEN BOTH JOIN TOGETHER IN MEAL PLANNING. TO FOLLOW PROPERLY, YOU MUST STAY FOCUSED!

RENAL AND DIABETES PATIENT DIET CALL FOR THE BEST YOU HAVE TO OFFER IN FOLLOWING AND DOING THE BEST YOU CAN IN MEAL PLANNING, PURCHASING YOUR FOODS, PREPPING, COOKING, AND THE WILLINGNESS TO SACRIFICE OLD AND FAMILIAR WAYS OF EATING. HERE ARE SOME OF THE FOODS BOTH DIETS CAN HAVE, PREPARED IN THE PROPER WAYS. AS YOU READ, A FEW WILL BE USED IN MEAL PLANNING. STEWS CAN BE MADE, PASTA COMBINATIONS, VEGGIE SOUPS, EGG OMELETS, SALADS, FRESH HOMEMADE BURGERS, UN-PROCESSED FRESH GROUND VARIETY OF MEATS, SMOOTHIES, VARIETY OF MEAT AND CHEESE SALADS, KEEP THE NON-DAIRY FOODS UP FRONT AND ALL OTHERS WAY BACK. ALTHOUGH EGGS AND MEAT COUNT PER SERVING COUNTS IN PROTEIN SOME UP THE SAME, THE TASTE IS DIFFERENT, SO I STAY WITHIN THE CORRECT PORTION AND ALLOWANCES. EATING UNHAPPILY, I IMAGINE, IS THE WORSE HURT CONCERNING FOOD ONE COULD HAVE. IF YOU ENJOY A LITTLE MEAT IN THE A.M. WITH YOUR EGG, OK JUST FOLLOW THE AMOUNT AND STAY FAR AWAY FROM PROCESSED MEATS. (THE ONLY WAY I SEE YOU BEING ABLE TO DO THIS IS TO HAVE HALF OF EACH UNLESS YOUR DIET ALLOWS YOU 2 MEATS AT BREAKFAST TIME.???

DO NOT START TAKING FOODS FROM ONE MEAL TO ANOTHER UNLESS YOU HAVE THE OK FROM YOUR

NUTRITION LEADER. STOP! SNEAKING AND HIDING WHAT YOU EAT THE SECRET WILL NOT LAST TOO LONG FROM YOUR HEALTHCARE TEAM. REMEMBER, THEY ARE READING THE SCALES AND BLOOD REPORTS SMILE. YOU ARE HARMING YOURSELF AND DELAYING YOUR WELLNESS. WE OFTEN TELL ROBERT WHAT WE DO NOT ALLOW YOU IS BECAUSE LOVE WILL NOT LET US TURN OUR HEADS TO THE WRONG YOU TRY TO HAVE AT TIMES, BEING HUMAN AND HAVING WANTS AND NEEDS WILL ALWAYS BE AROUND, WE HAVE A HEALTHY MEAL PLANNING REGIMEN, CHANGING THE FOOD CONTENT OFTEN. READ THE REPORTS SENT HOME WELL AND TRY HARD TO MAKE THE MISTAKES RIGHT THE NEXT TIME. BE SURE THE PATIENT READS IT ALSO WITH GREAT CONCERN. WHEN ROBERT'S REPORT ARRIVES, HE SAYS BEFORE HE HANDS IT TO ME, OH BOY, HERE SHE GOES. I WILL PREACH FOR A WHILE TO HIM IF THE REPORT IS BAD IN AN AREA. I KNOW FOR SURE IT SHOULD HAVE BEEN GOOD. WHEN YOU ARE NOT DEALING WITH MINORS BUT FULL GROWNUPS, THEY MUST TAKE CONSIDERATION FOR THEMSELVES FIRST. MAKE EACH DIFFICULT DAY TURN GOOD THE NEXT DAY, TRYING NEVER TO STOP. AS PEOPLE, WE CAN ONLY DO OUR BEST. TRY THE FOLLOWING DESSERTS.

FOR DIABETIC and RENAL

STRAWBERRY COOL CAKE

FRESH SLICED SWEETENED STRAWBERRIES OVER PLAIN VANILLA POUND CAKE (HOMEMADE) USE PORTION CONTROL WITH CAKE.

-1 TBSP. OF NONDAIRY WHIP CREAM ON TOP AND PLACE IN THE FRIDGE. LIGHTLY COVERED.

BAKED PEAR COOKIE DELIGHT

FRESH SLICED PEARS, NO SKIN, SHORT BREAD COOKIES SOAKED IN SOY ALMOND MILK. THEN WARMED.

APPLE CRISP

PEELED DICED SWEET APPLES, CINNAMON, SWEETENER, VANILLA, APPLE.

JUICE, BAKE, AND ENJOY. GARNISH WITH CORN CRUSHED FLAKES.

HONEY RICE PUDDING

COOKED WHITE RICE, EGGS, HONEY, NUTMEG, NUT FLAVORING (NO NUTS) STIR AND BAKE. USE SUGAR-FREE SYRUP IT DOES NOT TAKE BUT A SMALL AMOUNT, 1 TO 2 TABLESPOONS.

FRUIT CHILL DELIGHT

CHILLED WATERMELON AND WATER-PACKED FROZEN FRUITS APPROVED BY THE MEDICAL TEAM.

TOP WITH ONE JELL O CUBE.

WHEN USING FOODS LIKE FRESH FRUITS, BE AWARE THAT THEY ARE NATURALLY SWEETENED AND CARRY SUGAR IF SO, THAT MEANS CALORIES ARE INVOLVED.

JUST GO BY THE ALLOWED SERVING AMOUNTS. DO NOT OVERLOAD IT BECAUSE YOU CAN HAVE IT. THIS CAN BECOME AN ENEMY.

HAPPY CRISPY CAKES

COVER RICE CAKES WITH AN ASSORTMENT OF BABY DESSERTS, CHANGING DESSERTS OFTEN.

CHOOSE FROM A VARIETY OF BABY FRUITS AND DESSERTS THAT ARE OK ON YOUR DIET. GREAT HEALTHY CHOICES WHAT IS HEALTHIER THAN BABY FOODS?

ANY CHOICE IS GREAT ON A RICE CAKE. PURCHASE PLAIN AND UNSALTED.

***THIS IS A DIABETIC MEAL ONLY. ***

DIABETIC DIET

BREAKFAST

SMALL FRUIT JUICE

1 EGG/MARGARINE

HOT CEREAL

TOAST/SUGAR-FREE JAM

COFFEE OR TEA/ NON-DAIRY CREAM

LOW-FAT MILK

SUGAR SUB

MID-MORNING SNACK

WATER-PACKED CANNED FRUIT/PEANUT BUTTER CRACKERS.

LUNCH

LOW-FAT BEEF CAULIFLOWER SOUP

SLICE ROAST BEEF/ WITH

BOK CHOY/SLICED TOMATOES.

HORSERADISH/MAYONNAISE

FIG /APPLE DESSERT

LEMON TEA/SUGAR SUB

LOW-FAT MILK

MID DAY SNACK

JELL O/SHORT BREAD COOKIES (4)

DINNER

BAKED SALMON/LEMON/PARSLEY

BABY KALE

FLUFFY RICE

PICKLED BEETS

PINEAPPLE CHEESECAKE

HOT TEA/LEMON

NIGHT SNACK

½ TUNA SANDWICH FRUIT JUICE.

DESSERT

TO PREPARE THIS QUICK AND TASTY DIABETIC DESSERT. 1 SMALL SLICE ANGEL FOOD CAKE SPREAD WITH LIGHT CREAM CHEESE TOPPED WITH LOW SUGAR CRUSHED PINEAPPLES.

YOU HAVE 1 FRUIT, 1 BREAD, AND 1 FAT IF YOU ARE ALLOWED 1800 CALORIES OR MORE. THIS DESSERT IS EASILY MADE.

A GREAT REWARD FOR GOOD BEHAVIOR FOR MY HUBBY.

**REMEMBER TO ASK YOUR NUTRITION LEADER PERMISSION TO REMOVE AND

REPLACE YOUR FOODS. WE TRY TO KEEP ROBERT'S REMOVAL AND REPLACEMENTS IN THE SAME ERROR OF EATING**

YOU MUST STAY IN THE SAME FOOD GROUPS, REPLACE A VEGETABLE WITH ANOTHER VEGGIE, NOT WITH BREAD, MEAT, OR ANY OTHER GIVEN FOOD, IS HOW I DO IT. THIS IS A DIFFERENT DAY, AND THE RULES CHANGE. THIS IS WHY IT IS A MUST THAT YOU STAY CONNECTED TO YOUR LEADERS IN A HEALTHY.

THIS IS A SHARING BOOK, NOT A "ME" BOOK, DO NOT MISUNDERSTAND THE PURPOSE OF THE BOOK. YOU ONLY CAN COMMENT ON ANY SITUATION IF YOU ARE OR HAVE GONE THROUGH IT ALSO.

WHEN YOU DESIRE SOUPS WITH MEAT AND ARE NOT ALLOWED PURCHASE (BROTHS OF THE MEATS YOU ARE ALLOWED). I HAVE FOUND OTHER COUNTRIES' SPICES AND SOME FOODS ARE PARTICULARLY GOOD.

AN UNDERSTANDING OF NUTRITION MUST BE THERE FOR THE PATIENT TO GET THE BEST MEAL PLANNING. WHAT IS HEALTHIER (SLICED PEACH PIE OR FRESH PEACH)? AFTER READING THIS FAR, I ASSURE YOU HAVE THE CORRECT ANSWER.

FOLLOW ME, AND LET US START PUTTING IT ALL TOGETHER.

THE RENAL DIET IS JUST WHAT IT SAYS, WITH LOW SODIUM, PHOSPHORUS, POTASSIUM, AND SALT, ALERTNESS ALSO RESTRICTED FLUID INTAKE.

THE DIABETIC DIET IS AN APPROX... 1800 CALORIES, LOW CHOLESTEROL, AND LOW SODIUM.

Both diets are restricted to sodium and salt. This is how I write and look at it.

Renal/ low salt/ low Cholesterol/Diabetic

BREAKFAST

Fresh bunch grapes approx.-10

½ cup CREAM OF RICE CEREAL

4oz NON-DAIRY MILK

1 SCRAMBLED EGG

1 WHITE TOAST

UNSALTED MARGARINE 1tbsp

SUGAR-FREE JELLY

4 ounces brewed hot beverage (if allowed)

8 ounces of fluids were used.

We are using a liquid egg that shows yellow for the yolk but is not there.

SNACK- Graham crackers/baby cobbler

LUNCH

2 ounces SLICE DARK TURKEY (no skin)

HEARTS OF LETTUCE LEAVES

SLICE ONION/PARSLEY

ON WHITE SOFT ROLL/LIGHT MAYONNAISE

SUGAR-FREE/PEACH/APPLE/CHUTNEY

8OUNCES DIET 7UP

SUGAR SUB

UNSALTED SEASONINGS

SNACK-AROUND 2 PM

1-OUNCE EXTRA SHARP CHEESE, UNSALTED CRACKERS (5) 4 OUNCES COOL FRESH FLAVORED WATER.

** 12 OUNCES OF FLUIDS USED. **

DINNER

4 OUNCES LOW SALT BROTH

3-OUNCE BAKED COD FISH

1/2 CUP PASTA/UNSALTED MARGARINE

FROZEN COOKED MUSTARD GREENS

SM 1 ALL SLICE BLUEBERRY/ANGEL FOOD CAKE

4OUNCES FLAVORED BREWED TEA

NIGHT SNACK- 1/2 MEAT SANDWICH, SMALL PEAR, 4 OUNCES COLD WATER.

** 12 OZ. FLUID USED**

FLUID ALLOWANCES ARE MET FOR TODAY.

ALWAYS BE SURE WHEN A DIET IS LOW IN FAT AND CHOLESTEROL. MAKE IT HAPPEN, DO NOT IGNORE IT.

ALL OF YOU OUT THERE, CHECK YOURSELF, PULL IN THE REIGNS, LISTEN FIRST TO YOUR MEDICAL STAFF, FOLLOW THROUGH, AND MOST OF ALL, BELIEVE IN YOURSELF. PRESERVATION OF ONESELF IS A RESPONSIBILITY AND A BLESSING THAT HAS BEEN GIVEN TO ALL OF US.

IF YOU LIKE WHAT YOU HAVE READ. BE SURE YOUR DIETICIAN OR NUTRITIONIST DOES, ALSO. GOLD. IS 85% OUT OF 100% SATISFIED DAILY. HIS REPORTS SHOW THAT HE IS NOT VERY FAR AWAY FROM EATING GOLD. I HAVE MADE IT CLEAR THAT THIS IS THE WAY WE DO IT. EVERYONE IS DIFFERENT AND CALLS FOR DIVERSE WAYS AND MEANS. IF YOU ARE FORTUNATE TO UNDERSTAND THE BASICS OF ANYTHING, USUALLY THE REST WILL FOLLOW IF YOU TRY TO GRASP IT.

TIPS:

DIABETICS ARE OUT THERE.

FOLLOW YOUR CALORIES DAILY GIVEN BY YOUR MEDICAL STAFF.

TAKE YOUR GLUCOSE AND READ OFTEN DAILY.

WATCH CLOSELY FOR CUTS OR BRUISES AND REPORT RIGHT AWAY TO THE DOCTOR.

CARBS ARE NOT THE ONLY ENEMY IN DIABETES; FATS AND PROTEINS PLAY A PART ALSO.

STOP! ALLOWING FRIENDS AND FAMILY TO DIRECT YOU
UNLESS THEY HAVE BEEN PROVEN TO BE QUALIFIED.
FOLLOW THE PROPER PROCEDURES FOR A SICK
PERSON. LOOK! I FIND MYSELF DOING IT WITH MY
GROWN CHILDREN, SO IT DOES HAPPEN. THEY PUT ME
WHERE I SHOULD BE IN A MANNER AND PLEASANT
WAY. CHECK OUT THE ISSUE WITH YOUR DOCTOR'S
SMILE.

DIABETIC/RENAL/LOW-FAT

BREAKFAST

1 COOKED EGG WHITE

1/2 CUP CEREAL

1 SMALL FRESH FRUIT

1 TOAST/MARGARINE

4 OUNCES OF NON-DAIRY MILK

4 OUNCES BREWED COFFEE/SUGAR SUB.

MID-MORNING SNACK, 4 OUNCES SUGAR-FREE JELLO
TOPPED WITH 1 TABLESPOON CINNAMON
APPLESAUCE (NATURAL).

**12 OUNCES OF FLUID USED

JELL O IS ALSO FLUID IN THE BEGINNING AND END
MUST BE ACCOUNTED FOR.

MOST DIABETIC DIETS ARE CALCULATED TO OFFER 3
MEALS A DAY AND 3 SNACKS. FOLLOW YOURS.

Lunch

Assorted seafood salad bowl

2 can oysters.

1 boiled shrimp

Water-packed tuna fish.

5 Unsalted assorted bread sticks

1/2 cup fresh raspberries/whip cream

4 ounces of lime tea

Sugar sub.

Snack-

bunch grapes (12)

4 ounces of non-dairy milk

8 ounces were used.

Dinner

Steamed Duck (removed fat) with onions/rice.

Buttered corn

Sweet cabbage, carrot, veggie coleslaw

Small sourdough roll

Unsalted margarine

Sugar-free preserves

Hot beverage 8 ounces

HS snack (hours of sleep) cold cereal/ 4 ounces almond milk/fruit

32 ounces for the day

Quick but healthy snacking.

Unsalted popcorn/grated sharp cheese.

Graham cracker/applesauce dip.

Chilled watermelon/sweetened cranberries.

Sweetened cranberries overnight with sugar sub.

Celery stuffed- with light cream cheese(chilled)

Smoothie-4 ounces cranberry juice/4 ounces diet 7up/slice peaches water packed/grapes.

Place in a blender, then chill. Keep in your assigned group of fruits and fluids if cranberry juice is sugar-free both sides can enjoy my smoothie

ONLY 4 OUNCES of FLUIDS NECESSARY.

If you saddle up and just try, you can bring some awesome recipes for yourself. Remember, eating is a pleasure, not a torment. Because meals are met, does not mean the plans are

CORRECT. DO NOT EAT BECAUSE IT IS EXPECTED OF YOU. EAT BECAUSE WHAT YOU EAT, YOU INTEND TO ENJOY. JUST BECAUSE YOU BUY HEALTHY FOOD DOES NOT ALWAYS MEAN YOU ARE DOING IT CORRECTLY. PURCHASING THE SAME GROUP OF FOODS WEEK AFTER WEEK AND NEVER TRYING ANYTHING DIFFERENT IS NOT A GOOD STEP TOWARD HEALTHY.

YOU CAN ONLY GET ALL YOU NEED BY EATING A VARIETY OF DIFFERENT FOODS.

PINEAPPLE CHEESECAKE

WATER-PACKED PINEAPPLES/LIGHT CREAM CHEESE/ANGEL FOOD CAKE.

SPREAD CAKE WITH WHIP CREAM CHEESE AND ADD ON TOP PINEAPPLES. (QUICK AND GOOD) RENAL AND DIABETIC TREAT.

WHEN YOU CHOOSE CREAM CHEESE, PURCHASE FAT-FREE. KEEP WELL, THIS IS HOW OUR DAY IN EATING BEGINS AND ENDS. THERE ARE DAYS THAT WE STRAY, BUT NOT OFTEN. BAD MEAL PLANNING CAN DO HARM AND BE A BLOCKAGE FROM YOU GETTING TO YOUR RIGHT PLACE IN HEALTH AND HAPPINESS. MAKE SURE YOU USE THE AMOUNT OF FAT ALLOWED FOR DIABETICS, IF YOU WANT A SALAD WITH DRESSING AND A SPREAD FOR YOUR POTATOES OR VEGGIES, MAKE A HOMEMADE DRESSING OR PURCHASE WHAT I CALL A ZERO-CALORIE DRESSING. KEEP AN OPEN EYE ON MY WEBSITE FOR A COUPLE OF HOMEMADE RECIPES.

I FIND THE EXCHANGE SYSTEM, WHICH I CALL

REMOVALS AND REPLACEMENTS, WORKS WELL FORMED. I STAY IN THE SAME FOOD GROUPS WHEN I DO THIS, AND I TRY HARD NOT TO TAKE A PARTICULAR FOOD FROM ONE MEAL TO ANOTHER. YES, I DO SOMETIMES. FOR EXAMPLE, IF I DO NOT WANT MY FRUIT BUT JUICE OR BREAD FOR PASTA, STAYING IN THE SAME GROUP OF FOODS.

READERS, IF YOU ENJOYED AND RECEIVED SOME MOTIVATION OR UPLIFT IN GOING THIS WAY, DISCUSS IT WITH YOUR DIABETIC AND RENAL MEDICAL LEADERS. DON'T TAKE WHAT I SHARE IN ANY OF MY BOOKS AND RUN, DO WHAT I DO, AND CHECK ALWAYS WITH YOUR LEADERS FIRST. WE ALL ARE DIFFERENT AND HAVE TO BE TREATED DIFFERENTLY IN OUR HEALTH CONDITIONS, ALTHOUGH THEY MAY SEEM THE SAME. I FIND IT SO SAD TO HAVE TO KEEP SAYING THIS SO OFTEN WE ARE ALL VERY GROWN AND TO SAY WE DO NOT KNOW ANY BETTER IN THIS DAY AND TIME WITH FAMILIES YOUNG MIDDLE AGED AROUND US HELPING. TO GET A GOOD COMEBACK IN YOUR MEALS, JUST LEARN HOW BOTH DIETS WORK TOGETHER, FRIENDS. IF YOU DO NOT, YOUR GOAL WILL NEVER COME.

TIPS FOR YOU:

BE AWARE OF TOO MANY FLUIDS IF YOU HAVE BEEN TOLD TO.

FOLLOW ONLY THE GUIDELINES YOUR HEALTH PROFESSIONALS HAVE GIVEN TO YOU. IF CONFUSED, TALK WITH YOUR DIALYSIS TEAM ABOUT YOUR PROBLEMS.

THERE IS NO QUICK WAY OUT OF ANY ILLNESS, TIME, PATIENCE, AND, MOST OF ALL, FOLLOWING DIRECTIONS AT YOUR BEST. IT IS ABOUT YOU.

REMEMBER, THIS IS AN IMPORTANT AND SERIOUS CONDITION IF YOU MUST WORK EVERY DAY!

I TRY HARD WITH MY (WEB SITE)

WWW.OURSENIORHOOD.NET

TO HELP, IT TAKES MORE THAN ME. MONEY IS NOT THE QUESTION, OR ANSWER SHARING IS. YES, IT WILL BE HARDER TO DO MEAL PLANNING WHEN YOU HAVE MORE THAN ONE CONDITION, BUT YOU WILL IT TAKES TIME HOPEFULLY, IT WILL NOT TAKE TOO MUCH TIME. I WOULD ENJOY HELPING WHOEVER, BUT I CAN ONLY GO TO A CERTAIN LEVEL. MY AWESOME EXPERIENCES AND EDUCATION IN THIS AREA IS WHY I HAVE BUILT MY WEBSITE FOR ALL OF US. SMILE. NO CHARGES

Hope in sharing my outlook on two health conditions that seem to be on the very top of bad health list, will motivate, and help guide you in your journey through it all.

Diana

www.ingramcontent.com/pod-product-compliance
Lightning Source LLC
Chambersburg PA
CBHW072011280526
45788CB00013B/2535